WEIGHT FREE
WORKOUT

MEN'S HEALTH® BEST

WEIGHT-FREE WORKOUT

EDITED BY **JOE KITA**,
MEN'S HEALTH® MAGAZINE

This edition first published in 2005 by
Rodale International Ltd
7–10 Chandos Street
London
W1G 9AD
www.rodale.co.uk

© 2005 Rodale Inc.

"Men's Health®" is a registered trademark of Rodale Inc.

Interior photographs:
Beth Bischoff p. 31, 32, 37, 38, 39, 42, 43, 48, 49, 50, 51, 64, 66, 67, 68, 69, 70, 71, 74, 76, 79, 84, 85, 86, 87, 88, 90, 91, 92, 93, 94; Brand X Pictures p. 6, 33; Corbis p. 14, 21; Digital Vision p. 63; Todd France p. 34, 35, 40, 41; Svend Lindbaek p. 89; Michael Mazzeo p. 11, 22, 23, 24, 25, 26, 27, 28, 29, 30, 44, 45, 46, 47, 52, 53, 54, 55, 58, 59, 60, 61, 62, 65, 72, 73, 75, 77, 78, 80, 81, 82, 83; Photodisc p. 9, 16, 36

Printed and bound in the UK by CPI Bath using acid-free paper from sustainable sources.
1 3 5 7 9 8 6 4 2

ISBN 1-4050-7756-5

This paperback edition distributed to the book trade by Pan Macmillan Ltd

Notice
The information in this book is meant to supplement, not replace, proper exercise training. All forms of exercise pose some inherent risks. The editors and publisher advise readers to take full responsibility for their safety and know their limits. Before practising the exercises in this book, be sure that your equipment is well maintained, and do not take risks beyond your level of experience, aptitude, training and fitness.

The exercise and dietary programmes in this book are not intended as a substitute for any exercise routine or dietary regime that may have been prescribed by your doctor. As with all exercise and dietary programmes, you should get your doctor's approval before beginning.

Visit us on the Web at *www.menshealth.co.uk*

RODALE
LIVE YOUR WHOLE LIFE™

CONTENTS

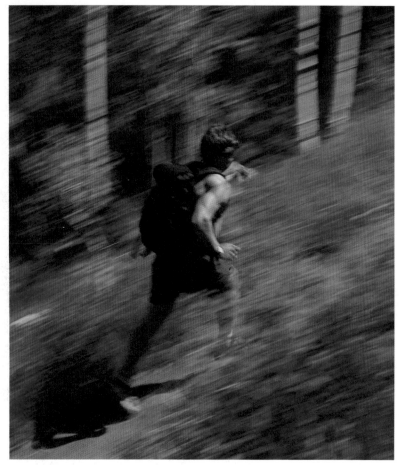

Most of your recreational activities don't involve weights – so knowing how to train without weights makes good sense.

INTRODUCTION

When we picture a modern-day workout we almost always picture a guy at the gym standing, sitting or lying down at a machine stacked with weights. Although there's no arguing that weight training can be an important part of any man's fitness routine, there are many practical reasons why a weight-free workout can be just as effective, serve as an occasional alternative to weights or actually be more beneficial for certain types of men, depending on their fitness goals.

4. **Latissimus dorsi**. The much-sought-after 'V' shape in the back comes from strong 'lats'. Pull-ups and chin-ups are great for working this group.

5. **Deltoids.** These muscles include the anterior deltoid, medial deltoid and posterior deltoid, and are located at the top of the shoulders. Press-ups and the Side Straddle Hop work the 'delts'.

6. **Biceps.** The front of the upper arms, the biceps group is the target of a lot of weight training, much of it superfluous. Any good exercise that involves the arms will work, but not overwork, the biceps.

7. **Triceps.** The back of the upper arm gets a good workout from a variety of press-ups.

8. **Gluteals.** The 'glutes' include the *gluteus maximus*, the muscle that covers your rear end. Lunges, squats, jumps, skips, step-ups and the Shuttle Run work the glutes.

FOLLOW THESE TWO SIMPLE EATING RULES

Finding time to exercise can be tough, especially when you have to adjust your workout to your eating schedule. Here's an easy-to-remember guide to pre- and post-exercise nutrition (for a detailed look at diet and nutrition, see page 16):

1. Don't eat a big meal less than an hour before you work out, but do try to get something down before you exercise. Grab a carb-protein shake 5 minutes before your workout and sip it throughout the session.

2. Eat carbohydrates and protein as soon as you can after your workout. The carbs help replace energy stores needed for your next workout; the protein repairs your muscles.

9. **Quadriceps.** The 'quads', a large muscle group, make up the front of the thigh. You'll work the quadriceps with lunges, squats, jumps, skips and step-ups.

10. **Hamstrings.** These large muscles run up the back of the thigh and need to be loose for almost any athletic activity. (You'll spend a good amount of time stretching your hamstrings before any workout.) Squats, jumps, skips, step-ups and the Shuttle Run especially target the hamstrings.

11. **Hip abductors and adductors.** These are the muscles of the inner and outer thigh. The abductors are located on the outside of your leg and move the leg away from the body. The adductors, located on the inside, pull the leg across the body. Exercises that work the hips include the Dirty Dog, Hip Adduction and Donkey Kick.

12. **Calf.** Located on the back of the lower leg, the calf muscles include the *gastrocnemius* and the *soleus*. The *gastrocnemius* gives the calf its rounded shape. The *soleus* runs under the *gastrocnemius*. As with the hamstrings, you should devote some time to stretching the calf muscles, which are especially targeted by jumps, squats, skips, step-ups and the Shuttle Run.

13. **Lower back.** The *erector spinae* muscles support the back and are responsible for good posture (remember to work them next time someone tells you to stand up straight). Squats and floor exercises work the lower back.

14. **Abdominals.** The 'abs' are made up of the *rectus abdominis*, which runs the length of the abdomen, and the external obliques, which are located on the sides and front of the abdomen. Crunches hit the *rectus abdominis*, and variations on the crunch such as twists work the external obliques. Boxing exercises such as the Horse-Stance Twist and 'Slip a Punch,' and floor exercises like the Curl-up also work the abs.

Workout Basics

It seems that anything worth doing is worth making incredibly complicated, especially workouts. We start adding exercises to hit every muscle from every angle; we run forwards, then backwards and sideways; we crunch, reverse crunch, side crunch and number crunch. Then we're so confused we forget why we were working out in the first place. Drop the calculator. It's time to make exercise simple again. Cut time, aggravation and wasted effort without sacrificing results. You'll enjoy your weight-free routine more and profit more from it – which is why you work out in the first place, right?

Time of Day. Research has consistently shown that exercising at the same time each workout day increases your chances of sticking with it. Pick the time you like. You may have heard that morning workouts are better, since testosterone levels are higher. Forget you heard that. Hormonal fluctuations are important, but they may not correlate to performance gains. The optimal time to work out is any time you can fit it into your schedule.

STRETCHING

Nobody wants to be called a stiff. 'Inflexible' and 'rigid' are just as undesirable. A stiff body is like a trial separation from your well-being. Tight hamstrings can lead to runner's knee. Tight pectorals limit your strength and put your shoulders at risk of injury. We've included a number of vital stretches as part of the weight-free workout. Spend twice as much time stretching your tight muscles as your flexible muscles. You should focus on problem areas instead of muscles that are already flexible. If you're under 40, hold your stretches for 30 seconds. If you're over 40, hold them for 60 seconds. As you reach your 40s, your muscles become less pliable, so they need to be stretched for longer.

Swimming builds endurance, muscle strength and cardiovascular fitness without stressing your body.

Keep a Calendar. Do the workout, and then cross it off. Mark an 'X' on your calendar on the days you exercise. A recent study found that exercisers who used this simple system of tracking workouts made more progress than those who didn't.

Stick With It. Stay with an exercise programme until it stops working for you. Switching too often from one programme to the next can get in the way of your goals. You'll make your workouts simpler (and see better results) if you stick to one programme for six to 12 weeks, or until it stops working. Is it working?

Two benchmarks: your waist tightens while your strength improves.

One at a Time. Do one exercise for each muscle group. Unless you're a bodybuilder, there's no need to hit a muscle from every conceivable angle each time you train it. Work hard on one or two exercises per muscle group.

Set a Time Limit. Forget the hours of working out you imagine other guys are doing. Aim for one hour. The dropout rate for routines that last more than 60 minutes is high. At one hour, your body slows down its production of muscle-building hormones and cranks up the stress hormone cortisol, which can have a testosterone-blocking, muscle-wasting effect.

Recover Faster. A lot of people adopt a weight-free workout because they've sustained an injury that requires a low-impact fitness routine. If you're recovering from a muscle injury, begin exercising again as soon as you can. Try a few minutes at low intensity to test yourself. Go slowly – no explosive movements. If you experience pain, stop immediately. Afterwards, ice the area for 20 minutes and exercise again the next day. You should be able to go a little harder and longer each workout.

Reach Your Goals. Set your goals in reverse. That is, pick a date of completion and work backwards, writing down short-term goals as you go. The goals then seem more like deadlines.

Stay Hydrated. Start the day with a full litre bottle of water. Finish it off by the end of the day. Along with other beverages like milk and juice, that should keep you hydrated. Alcohol doesn't count – it not only makes you sprint to the urinal, it takes some of your body's own water out, too.

Drinking too much alcohol can lower your testosterone levels and decrease overall muscle mass. However, drinking moderately (two drinks or fewer per day) won't harm testosterone levels and can actually improve your cardiovascular health.

Sleep. Depriving yourself of sleep not only limits your ability to grow muscle – your body releases most of its growth hormone while you sleep – but also severely impairs your co-ordination and mental focus. This translates to less strength and a greater chance of injuring yourself. If you work out, you should sleep for the optimum amount of time each night – at least seven or eight hours a night for most guys. If you have to go a few nights with limited sleep, don't count on giving your best performance.

Diet and Nutrition

You're going to get hungry every two to three hours, guaranteed. Whatever your fitness goals, whatever the frequency and intensity of your workouts, the key to diet and nutrition is: be prepared. If you know you're going to be away from decent food, take some healthy snacks with you. Nuts and dried fruit are easy and compact, and require no special preparation or refrigeration. If you need to pack something more meal-like, try a peanut butter and jam sandwich on multigrain bread. Keep apples nearby everywhere you go; if you eat one apple a day, the pectin will keep you too full to crave anything that's really bad for you.

Protein

A recent study compared high carbohydrate with high protein diets for weight loss in extremely overweight men. Even though the calories were the same, the high protein group lost 28 per cent more weight in the four week study. More importantly, the metabolic rates of the men in the high protein group were 14 per cent faster than the others. You need no more than 1.5 grams of protein per kilogram of body weight (that's just less than one gram per pound). Any excess will be stored as fat.

Add the right exercises to your weight-loss plan to ensure you don't diet away all that hard-earned muscle.

If you find it difficult to eat foods that are high in protein, protein supplements are a possible option, but they can be expensive. A single serving of a typical supplement contains between 18 and 40 grams of protein. All are sweetened with a sugar called maltodextrin, so you don't have to add anything but water and then mix them up in a shaker or blender. Two servings can supply your daily protein allowance.

Protein bars are another alternative, with one minor drawback. Many are made with chemicals called sugar alcohols and too much of these in your system can lead to serious flatulence. You shouldn't experience this problem if you keep your intake to one bar a day – but consider yourself warned.

Carbohydrates

The best carbohydrates for your metabolism are those with a low glycaemic index. The glycaemic index measures how fast your body processes a food. Foods with a high index (such as white bread and highly-processed breakfast cereals) make you hungrier faster.

Unfortunately, there's nothing intuitive about the glycaemic index. Many people consider pasta to be a fast-acting carbohydrate, but most pastas fall in the middle of the range. Likewise a high-fibre cereal like All Bran is mid-range.

In other words, if you want to use the glycaemic index, you have to spend time memorizing it or use a cheat sheet. The box below shows how to replace five common foods

GLYCAEMIC SWAP LIST

Foods with a low glycaemic index are slow burners, so they'll keep you full longer. A simple rule for slowing your body's response to food, no matter how high the glycaemic index, is to add protein, fat and/or fibre to any meal. The glycaemic index numbers following the foods in this chart are based on a scale on which pure glucose has a score of 100. The higher the number, the faster the food burns.

Instead of...	Try...
White bread (70)	Multigrain bread (48)
Corn flakes (83)	All Bran or porridge (42)
Baked potato (85)	Low-carb pasta (27)
Watermelon (72)	Pear (37)
Chocolate-caramel bar (64)	Peanut-based sweets (32)

SOURCES OF PROTEIN

Food	Protein (grams)
170 g can of tuna	39
1 medium (130 g, cooked weight) chicken breast	34
2 thick slices (90 g, cooked weight) lean roast beef	26
roast beef sandwich	22
6 egg whites	18
turkey sandwich on wholemeal bread	18
2 whole eggs	13
small bag (50 g) cashews	10
4 tbsp (160 g) baked beans	8
150 g container low-fat yogurt	8
240 ml skimmed milk	8
small portion (200 g, cooked) spaghetti	7
30 g oatmeal (uncooked)	4

with a high glycaemic index with others that are lower on the list.

Perfect Meal Timing

If you want to understand energy balance in an instant, think of your body as a car that operates 24 hours a day. You would never expect your car to get you from one place to the next without systematic refuelling, just as you know there's no point in putting more petrol in the tank than it's designed to hold, but that's how many of us operate our bodies. We try to run on empty for hours, then dump in more fuel than we can handle. This strategy is self-destructive.

Let's say you really want to lose fat and decide to jog first thing in the

morning on an empty stomach. The easiest way to get energy is to break down muscle mass. Your body can convert specific amino acids – the building blocks of muscle – to glucose, the sugar that powers human activity. Someone running before eating may actually be breaking down the very tissue he's trying to improve. This is counterproductive – a 'muscle-loss' diet.

The 'fat-gain' diet is probably more typical of most of us. With this one, you wait a long time between meals and then, when you're ravenously hungry, you wipe out a whole buffet table. This guarantees that you'll get a larger surge of the hormone insulin than you ordinarily would and that means more fat storage.

You can probably combine the 'muscle-loss' and 'fat-gain' strategies mentioned above to turn your body into a perfect muscle-burning, fat-storing machine. Hard exercise slows down appetite in the short term, but as you get used to it, your appetite matches your exertion level. So you go out and run 10 kilometres on an empty stomach, then eat enough to fuel a 15-kilometre run; the net effect is that you've lost muscle on the run and gained fat from the post-run meal. Energy balance is the answer:

- Eat as soon as you wake up.

- Make sure you eat a small meal before you exercise, no matter what time of day it is. Not only does the food prevent

your muscle tissue from becoming cardio fuel, it also increases the number of calories you burn during and after exercise. Studies show that exercise following a meal enhances metabolism.

- Eat immediately after exercising, when your body has depleted its energy reserves. Act fast or you'll start burning muscle for energy.

- Eat a total of five to six small meals each day. Studies have shown that athletes who added three daily snacks to their three square meals lost fat and gained muscle, as well as improving in all the other things that are important to athletes, such as

SHAKE YOUR MUSCLES

Eat immediately after your workout. A recent Danish study (the country, not the pastry) found that older men who drank a shake with 10 grams of protein, 7 grams of carbohydrate and 3 grams of fat (about the same as in a 240 ml (8 fl oz) glass of milk) within five minutes after their weight workout gained muscle, but men who consumed the drink two hours later did not. For a serious post-workout muscle-building shake, try this formula:

Blend two medium scoops of fat-free or low-fat frozen chocolate yogurt, 4 tbsp of egg substitute, 240 ml (8 fl oz) of skimmed milk, a large banana and a tablespoon of unsweetened cocoa powder, and drink. You'll down 23 grams of protein, 52 grams of carbs and only four grams of fat.

WORKOUT MEAL PLAN

Use this great meal-planning system when your exercise affects what you should eat, and when you should eat it.

IF YOU WORK OUT IN THE MORNING

Meal 1: PRE-WORKOUT SNACK

- 150 ml (5 fl oz) whey protein shake (or)
- banana and hard-boiled egg (or)
- cereal with skimmed milk

Meal 2: BREAKFAST
(Immediately following workout)

- egg-white omelette with vegetables (or)
- bowl of porridge
- orange juice

Meal 3: MID-MORNING SNACK

- yogurt and fruit (or)
- 300 ml (10 fl oz) whey protein shake and fruit

Meal 4: LUNCH

- salad with grilled chicken and olive oil dressing (or)
- tuna or ham sandwich on wholemeal bread

Meal 5: MID-AFTERNOON SNACK

- unsalted peanuts or cashews and an apple (or)
- meal-replacement bar (or)
- low-fat yogurt

Meal 6: DINNER

- grilled salmon, chicken breast or sirloin steak
- green salad with olive oil dressing

IF YOU WORK OUT AT LUNCH

Meal 1: BREAKFAST

- scrambled eggs with wholemeal toast (or)
- porridge with crushed flaxseeds (linseeds) and yogurt

Meal 2: MID-MORNING/PRE-WORKOUT SNACK
(No more than one hour before workout)

- 300 ml (10 fl oz) whey protein shake with fruit

Meal 3: LUNCH
(Immediately following workout)

- chicken breast and salad in a wholemeal roll
- fruit

Meal 4: MID-AFTERNOON SNACK

- unsalted peanuts or cashews and an apple (or)
- meal-replacement bar (or)
- hard-boiled egg

Meal 5: DINNER

- Hamburger made with ground sirloin (90% lean) or turkey on wholemeal bun
- cucumber and tomato salad drizzled with olive oil

IF YOU WORK OUT AFTER WORK

Meal 1: BREAKFAST

• scrambled eggs with wholemeal toast (or)
• wholegrain cereal with blueberries and skimmed milk

Meal 2: MID-MORNING SNACK

• 300 ml (10 fl oz) whey protein shake with peanut butter (or)
• yogurt and cashews

Meal 3: LUNCH

• chicken breast
• steamed vegetables
• wholemeal roll

Meal 4: MID-AFTERNOON SNACK

• unsalted peanuts or cashews and an apple (or)
• meal-replacement bar (or)
• cooked chicken leg

Meal 5: PRE-WORKOUT SNACK

• 150 ml (5 fl oz) whey protein shake

Meal 6: DINNER

• grilled salmon, chicken breast or sirloin steak
• green salad with olive oil dressing
• wild rice

power and endurance. Of course, you can't simply add a few hundred calories to your diet and lose weight, but you can redistribute your daily calories so you're eating more often but consuming less at individual meals.

• Eat before bed. If you're trying to build muscle and lose fat, you may need to eat a snack right before bed to keep your body from breaking down muscle tissue as you sleep. Planning this snack will help you resist the temptation to inhale an entire chocolate cake at midnight.

However you do it, it's clear that the worst dieting strategy is cutting out tons of calories indiscriminately in the hope of sudden dramatic weight loss. If you're more patient and try to lose half a kilogram (about one pound) a week every week or two, you'll be more likely to reach your goals and less likely to regain the unwanted weight.

The Benefits of Stretching

Some men are so pressed for time that they just want to get their workout over with as quickly as possible. They want to get right into it without warming up or stretching before they begin. But just a few minutes of stretching can be enormously beneficial to your workout. Just five to seven minutes of stretching before and after exercise will increase flexibility. Stretching may help to prevent injury and soreness, helps free your body of muscular tension, improves circulation and enhances muscle tone – giving your muscles a more defined look.

UPPER-BACK STRETCH

Hold your arms straight out in front of your chest and clasp your hands together. Push your arms forwards, rounding your shoulders and upper back. Hold for 10 seconds.

CHEST STRETCH

Clasp your hands together, palms up, behind your lower back. Pull your arms up towards your head. Hold for 10 seconds. Feel the stretch in the front of your chest and shoulders.

SHOULDER AND NECK STRETCH

Place both arms behind your back and grab your right wrist with your left hand. Tilt your head to the left and pull your right arm to the left. Hold for 10 seconds, then repeat on the other side.

HOW OFTEN SHOULD I STRETCH?

If you're stuck behind a desk all day, stretch every few hours to avoid back and shoulder tightness that comes from hunching over a keyboard. Do the Chest Stretch on page 23 to open your chest and relax your shoulders and back. To stretch your glued-to-the-chair glutes, cross your left leg over your right, resting your left ankle on your right knee. Bend forwards at the waist and hold the stretch for 10 seconds. Then switch legs and repeat.

POSTERIOR SHOULDER STRETCH

Grab the back of your left upper arm with your right hand and pull it across your chest gently. Hold for 10 seconds, then repeat on the other side.

Towel Stretch Circuit

Your muscles, like a good after-dinner glass of brandy, work best when warm. That's why you can do more challenging stretches at the end of a workout without much risk of injury.

HAMSTRING STRETCH

Lie on your back on the floor. Lift your legs, wrap the towel behind your thighs and gently pull your hamstrings and gluteals into a deeper stretch by pulling the ends of the towel. Hold for 15 to 30 seconds.

CHEST AND SHOULDER STRETCH

Now stand up, with the towel in your hands behind you. Bend forwards as you reach back with your arms, slowly stretching out your chest and shoulders. Hold this position for 15 to 30 seconds.

WARM MUSCLES WORK BETTER

When muscles are cold, they're stiffer. Light exercise before stretching warms them and makes them more pliable, improving the stretch and reducing the risk of muscle strain. Keep it simple – walk or slowly jog for 10 minutes to prepare your muscles for the exercises ahead.

TRICEPS STRETCH

Finally, hold one end of the towel in your right hand and lift your right arm over your right shoulder, so the towel hangs down your back. Reach up behind you with your left hand and grab the other end of the towel. Gently pull your triceps and lats into a deeper stretch. Hold for 15 to 30 seconds, then repeat on the other side.

LYING ILIOTIBIAL BAND STRETCH

The iliotibial band extends from the thigh down to and over the knee. It helps stabilize the knee during running and walking. This stretch will help prevent injury. Lie on your back. Keep your left leg straight and lift it across your body. Hold for 10 seconds. Repeat with the other leg.

BE FLEXIBLE

Flexibility is the easiest fitness element to develop. As with other types of training, improvement in flexibility depends on subjecting muscles to more than they're accustomed to by working them through a range of motion in a controlled and systematic way. You merely need to add 10 extra minutes or so to what you already do.

MODIFIED HURDLER STRETCH

Sit on the floor with your left leg straight out in front of you. Place your right foot flat against your left thigh. Bend forwards towards your left knee and hold for 10 seconds. Repeat with your right leg straight.

GROIN STRETCH

Sit on the floor and place the soles of your feet together. Grasp your ankles and gently push your knees down with your elbows. Hold for 10 seconds.

CALF STRETCH

From a standing position, step 60 centimetres forwards with your left foot and bend your right knee. Bend at the waist, grab the front of your left foot and pull it gently upwards. (If necessary, place your free hand on a chair or wall for balance.) Hold for 10 seconds. Switch sides and then repeat.

Full-Body Flexibility

Flexibility doesn't have to mean stretching and yoga and inner peace. It can mean sweat and grunts and a heart-pounding workout. These moves will stretch your muscles in ways that will help you with real-world activities, like starting a lawn mower. Perform these exercises as a circuit – one set of each stretch immediately after the other – as fast as possible. Do four or five circuits, 20 repetitions of each exercise. Two or three circuits is a good warmup for sports or weight lifting.

ROTATIONAL PRESS

Targets: Shoulders, Abdominals, Obliques, Gluteals, Calves, Ankles

Lift your right arm as high as you can above your shoulder and twist your body 90 degrees to the left, lifting your right heel as you turn. Then lower your right arm and raise your left arm as you twist to the right.

ALTERNATING UPRIGHT ROW

Targets: Lower Back, Chest, Obliques

Bend over slightly at the hips until your upper body is at a 30-degree angle. Look at the floor and let your arms hang straight down from your shoulders. Then lift your left elbow as high as possible, as if starting a lawn mower. As you lower your left arm, repeat the movement with your right arm.

REACHING LATERAL LUNGE

Targets: Lower Back, Gluteals, Hamstrings

Step to the left with your left leg, keeping the toes of your left foot pointing forwards. Bend your left knee about 20 degrees and lean over to touch the toes of your left foot with the fingertips of both hands. Push back to the starting position, then reach as high as you can with both hands. Repeat the movement to your right side. That's one repetition.

PART II:
Ultimate Workouts

THE 15-MINUTE WORKOUT

Go to Extremes

The following three-step programme might not be a 15-minute workout the first time you try it. It may take a few weeks to build up to that. Once you reach that point, you can add weight to make the moves even more difficult, try the exercises from different angles or invent your own exercises using the techniques described here. Do this workout 3 days in a row, rest a day, then do it 2 more days, before resting for 2 days. Repeat for the rest of your life, if you want.

EXTREME-RANGE ONE-LEG SQUAT

Targets: Quadriceps, Gluteus Maximus
Time: 5 Minutes

■ Stand with your back to a box, place your right foot on it and squat down. Hold for 2 seconds then release.

② Now, squat down further and hold the position as long as you can bear the burn. Repeat until your leg can't take it any more. Then repeat with your left foot on the box.

EXTREME-RANGE PULL-UP

Targets: Biceps, Latissimus Dorsi, Trapezius
Time: 5 Minutes

1 Using an overhand grip with your arms just beyond shoulder width, hang from a pull-up bar for 2 seconds. Drop from the bar and relax.

2 Now grab the bar again and hang as long as you can. Drop and rest a minute, then go up and hold again. Repeat until your back refuses to do any more.

EXTREME-RANGE PRESS-UP

Targets: Biceps, Latissimus Dorsi, Trapezius
Time: 5 Minutes

1 Set two sturdy boxes 75–85 centimetres apart. Drop into a press-up position and lower your chest between the boxes for 2 seconds.

2 Relax, then repeat, holding as long as you can. Rest a minute, then go down and hold again. Repeat until your upper body begs for mercy.

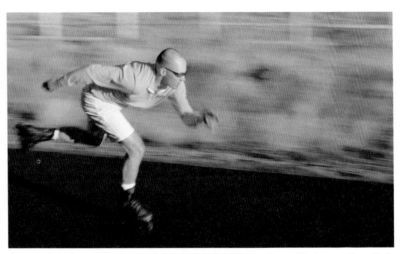

Strong lower-back muscles and powerful abdominals that stabilize your torso will help prevent lower-back strain when you rollerblade.

Save Your Back in 7 Minutes

Here is a back-saving programme that not only relieves current back pain, but also reduces your chances of a future back attack. This quick and easy four-exercise circuit is designed to increase back strength and flexibility through endurance-building movements that will help stabilize your back muscles. The result: strong, supple back muscles that will support you during any activity – anytime, anywhere.

YOUR WORKOUT SCHEDULE

Do the workout once a day, every day. You don't need rest days between lower-back workouts, since the idea is to build endurance, rather than strength. Plus, by performing these exercises daily, you'll strengthen your spine-stabilizing muscles. Perform the exercises as a circuit, doing them consecutively without rest in between.

CURL-UP

Targets: Whole Abdominal Region

1 Lie face-up on the floor with your left leg straight and flat on the floor. Your right knee should be bent and your right foot flat. Place your hands palms down on the floor underneath the natural arch in your lower back (don't flatten your back).

2 Slowly raise your head and shoulders off the floor without bending your lower back or spine and hold this position for 7 to 8 seconds, breathing deeply the whole time.

3 That's one repetition. Do four repetitions, then switch legs so that your right leg is straight and your left is bent.

TRAINER'S TIPS

- This exercise forces you to work all of your abdominal muscles while keeping your lower back in its naturally arched position. The move minimizes stress on your spine while increasing the endurance of the muscles.

- For a more challenging workout, try raising your elbows off the floor as you curl up, or begin the movement by contracting your abs and then curl up against that force.

CAT-CAMEL

Targets: Trapezius, Pectorals, Spinal Erectors

1 Get down on your hands and knees with your hands shoulder-width apart. Slowly lower your head between your arms as you push up as high as you can with your back, rounding your spine.

2 When you reach the top of the movement, slowly lower your back as you lift your head up, extend your neck forwards and up and arch your lower back by moving your belly button towards the floor.

3 That's one repetition. Do five to eight repetitions.

POSTURE IS KEY

The most dangerous position for your spine is fully flexed, or bent forwards like the letter C. Avoid that position by keeping your lower back in its naturally arched alignment in any exercise that requires you to bend over. Back injuries are common, but can be avoided through care and practice.

SIDE BRIDGE

Targets: Lateral Stabilizers

1️⃣ Lie on your left side with your knees straight and your upper body propped up on your left elbow and forearm. Place your right hand on your left shoulder and slowly raise your hips until your body forms a straight line from your shoulders to your knees.

2️⃣ Hold this position for 7 to 8 seconds, breathing deeply the whole time. Do four or five repetitions, then switch to your right side.

BIRD DOG

Targets: Lower- and Middle-Back Extensors

1️⃣ Get down on your hands and knees with your palms flat on the floor, shoulder-width apart. Slowly raise and straighten your right leg and left arm at the same time. Hold that position for 7 to 8 seconds, breathing deeply throughout the exercise.

2️⃣ Lower your arm and leg straight down and then sweep them along the floor back into the starting position.

3️⃣ That's one repetition. Perform four repetitions, then switch sides.

TRAINER'S TIP

This exercise works your lower- and middle-back extensors – the muscles that help you bend backwards – while producing half the stress on your spine that conventional back-extension exercises create.

THE 15-MINUTE WORKOUT

Shadowbox For Ripped Abs

Boxers can tell you that great abs don't just look good: these muscles contract to protect your internal organs from body shots and help you twist or lean to one side or the other to dodge fists or feet. That's why these modified boxing and martial-arts moves will help you build killer abs.

EXHALE AND CLENCH

Targets: Lateral Stabilizers
Time: 5 Minutes

1. Stand in a boxing pose (one foot slightly in front of the other, hands up) and imagine that you're absorbing a series of hits to the stomach.
2. Exhale and pull your belly in on each imagined strike.
3. Release your abdominal muscles and repeat.

TRAINER'S TIP

This exercise is great for your *transverse abdominis*, the strip of muscle that supports your internal organs and flattens your waistline.

HORSE-STANCE TWIST

Targets: Obliques, Abdominals
Time: 5 Minutes

1 Stand with your feet just slightly beyond shoulder-width apart, toes pointed forwards, knees bent at about a 60-degree angle, back straight, abs tight, hands up in a fighting posture.

2 Turn your torso to your left, pivoting on the balls of your feet if you need to (it's best to do this on an uncarpeted floor).

3 Feel the squeeze in the sides of your waist, then repeat to your right.

SLIP A PUNCH

Targets: Obliques, Abdominals
Time: 5 Minutes

1 Start in the same position as the Horse-Stance Twist, only stand more upright, with your hands at your sides.

2 Imagine a punch is coming right at your nose (or get a trusted friend to actually throw one). Lean to the left just far enough to elude the punch. Don't move anything but your upper torso.

3 Feel that contraction on the left side of your waist? Now dodge a punch by leaning in the other direction.

Six-Pack Isolation

The exercises in this simple gut-busting workout are specifically designed to exhaust the oblique muscles first so your *rectus abdominis* – the six-pack – is isolated later. Perform this workout as a circuit, with no rest between exercises. Do three circuits, resting 60 seconds after each.

MODIFIED BICYCLE KICK

Targets: Obliques, Rectus Abdominis

1. Lie on the floor with your hands behind your head, your right leg straight and off the floor. Bend your left leg so your knee is pulled towards your chest.

2. Lift your shoulder blades off the floor and take a count of two to touch your right elbow to your left knee. Pause, lower your elbow and shoulder blades back to the floor (again to a count of two), then immediately repeat the move on the other side – bringing your left elbow to your right knee and straightening your left leg.

3. Complete 15 repetitions on each side and then immediately do a set of 30 conventional crunches.

REVERSE CRUNCH

Targets: Rectus Abdominis

1 Lie face-up on the floor with your arms straight above you or braced on the sides of a doorway. Bend your knees and lift your heels off the floor and towards your buttocks.

2 Roll your hips up, bringing your knees towards your chest. As your lower back rises off the floor, straighten your legs, point your toes to the ceiling and lift your hips. Pause, then slowly reverse the motion. Do 20 repetitions.

ROLL UP

Targets: Rectus Abdominis

1 Lie face-up on the floor with your legs straight and your arms at your sides.

2 Push your heels into the ground and slowly lift your shoulders and back off the floor. Pause when your upper body is perpendicular to the floor, then slowly lower your body to a count of five. Perform 10 repetitions.

THE 20-MINUTE WORKOUT

Sculpt Olympian Legs

The exercises in this circuit will help you build overall leg strength, flexibility and endurance. If you're a beginner or haven't worked out for six months, do the moves as your lower-body workout and use only your body weight for each exercise. If you already work your legs weekly, incorporate these exercises into the beginning of your workout, but keep the weight light – 3- or 5-kilogram dumbbells, for instance. Do the workout two or three times a week, with at least a day of rest between sessions. Perform three sets of 10 to 14 repetitions of each move; for the step-ups, that means 10 to 14 with each leg.

FRONT STEP-UP

Targets: Quadriceps, Hamstrings, Gluteals
Time: 5 Minutes

1 The step should be high enough that your thigh is parallel to the floor when your foot is on the step.

2 Place your left foot on the step and push yourself up until your left leg is straight. Your right foot doesn't need to rest on the step.

3 Step back down, right foot first, followed by your left.

LATERAL STEP-UP

Targets: Groin, Quadriceps, Hamstrings, Gluteals, Calves
Time: 5 Minutes

1. Use a step that's about 30 centimetres high.
2. Follow the same procedure as for the Front Step-up, but stand sideways next to the step instead of facing it.

TRAINER'S TIPS

- Stand as straight as possible. This minimizes stress on the lower back and legs.

- Be certain to do the same number of repetitions for each foot. You can either alternate legs or complete a given number with one side, then switch to the other.

BELT SQUAT

Targets: Quadriceps, Hamstrings, Gluteals, Outer Thighs
Time: 5 Minutes

1 Stand with your hands behind your head and your knees slightly bent. Position a bungee cord just above your knees and push out as you squat.

2 Keep your body as upright as possible throughout the movement, and lower yourself until your thighs are parallel to the floor, then return to a standing position.

TRAINER'S TIP

Pushing out on the bungee cord with your outer-thigh muscles forces your adductors (inner-thigh muscles) to work harder to keep you stabilized.

BALL SQUAT

Targets: Quadriceps, Hamstrings, Gluteals, Inner Thighs
Time: 5 Minutes

1. Stand with your hands behind your head and your knees slightly bent. Hold a medicine ball or a basketball between your knees.

2. Keep your upper body as straight as possible and lower yourself until your thighs are parallel to the floor, then return to a standing position.

TRAINER'S TIP

Squeezing the ball with your adductors makes your abductors (outer thigh muscles) work overtime to help with your balance.

THE ULTIMATE POWER MOVE

If you aren't doing squats in your workout, then you don't have a workout. Squats shape the body and develop performance power – they're easy to learn and produce quick, dramatic results in both muscle size and strength.

To get the most out of each and every squat you do, focus on squatting deeper. The key is to descend until your thighs are parallel to the floor, while still keeping your heels on the floor and maintaining the natural arch in your lower back. This deeper squat builds muscle faster and is safer for your knees than a squat in which you stop before your thighs are parallel to the floor. When you cut a squat short like that, you turn your knees into brakes and you know what happens to brakes: they wear out.

THE 20-MINUTE WORKOUT

Lower-Body Beach Blast

Next time you head to the beach, you can get a great lower-body workout before you brave the waves and bathe in the sun. How? The secret is written in the sand. Sand provides less stability, making the simplest movements much harder. Don't go for the compacted sand near the water, which is too hard on the ankles. Find a soft, flat area, take off your shoes and do two sets of each exercise, with a minute of rest between exercises. Repeat the circuit, reapply your sunscreen and enjoy the rest of your day at the beach!

SHUTTLE RUN

Targets: Quadriceps, Calves, Hamstrings, Gluteals
Time: 5 Minutes

1 Make three parallel lines in the sand, 4.5 metres apart. Straddle the middle line with your knees slightly bent and your arms bent so your hands are in front of your thighs.

2 Move to your right and bend at the knees to touch the line with your right hand, then run to the left and touch the far left line with your left hand.

SAND SKIP

Targets: Quadriceps, Calves, Hamstrings, Gluteals
Time: 5 Minutes

1 Skip forwards so that you're jumping and landing on the same foot.

2 Work on leaping as high as possible by driving your knee upwards as you push off the ground with your opposite foot. Do five skips on each leg.

SQUAT JUMP

Targets: Quadriceps, Calves, Hamstrings, Gluteals
Time: 5 Minutes

1. Stand with your feet slightly more than shoulder-width apart and your fingers laced behind your head.

2. Bend at the knees to lower yourself until your thighs are at least parallel to the sand, then jump up as high as you can.

3. Sink directly into the next squat without pausing. Do a total of five repetitions.

TRAINER'S TIP

Don't have a beach handy? You can still do the workout, but take care to protect your knees. Try to do these moves on a carpeted or padded surface; a wooden aerobics studio floor is ideal.

JUMP AND STICK

Targets: Quadriceps, Calves, Hamstrings, Gluteals
Time: 5 Minutes

[1] Stand with your feet about shoulder-width apart, hands beside your thighs.

[2] Jump straight up, then land on only one leg with your knees bent, your shoulders slightly forwards and your buttocks and hips back. Your hands can end up slightly out to your sides and in front of you for balance.

[3] Try to steady yourself for 2 seconds, then return to the starting position and jump again. Alternate the leg you land on and do four jumps on each leg.

Balancing Act

Build Lower-body Endurance

To truly excel in your sport of choice, you need balance, endurance and strength. Whether you're racing down the football pitch or reaching for that seemingly impossible tennis shot, the ability to balance on a single leg, quickly change direction and start and stop your motion with the snap of a finger is definitely an asset. Here's a circuit that will improve your balance and quicken your step. Warm up for 5 minutes, then do these exercises, with only a minute of rest after each.

SINGLE-LEG BALANCE SQUAT

Targets: Quadriceps, Gluteals

1. Stand on a block or step (start with one that's about 15 centimetres high) and move one foot off the edge.

2. Bend the knee of the supporting leg so that the non-supporting foot brushes the floor. Hold that position for 3 to 5 seconds and then stand back up.

TRAINER'S TIP

When you can comfortably perform 20 balance squats, it's time to up the stakes and make this move more challenging – increase the height of the block (or step) to further develop your balance, endurance and coordination.

SINGLE-LEG SKI SQUAT

Targets: Quadriceps, Gluteals

1 Stand on one leg and place the other leg in front of you with your heel about 15 centimetres above the floor.

2 Squat down until the thigh of your back leg is almost parallel to the floor. Do 10 repetitions. Rest 15 seconds, then switch legs.

TRAINER'S TIP

If you're struggling to keep your balance, use two sturdy chairs for support until you feel comfortable with the move.

DOUBLE-LEG SKI SQUAT

Targets: Quadriceps, Gluteals

1 Lean against a wall, with your feet about 60 centimetres away from it and shoulder-width apart.

2 Bend your knees slightly and hold that position for 5 to 10 seconds. Bend deeper and hold.

3 Repeat until you've hit five different positions; go as low as you can without losing your balance. Work up to 30 seconds in each position.

Isoexplosion

2 Power Moves for Total Body Training

You live in the real world; you're going to miss some workouts. But when there's no equipment at hand, you can rely on isoexplosive training. Using only your body weight to maintain muscle, you'll be able to work out when you're on the road, stuck in the office or just unable to find your dumbbells. Try these two exercises for an intense full-body workout – any time, anywhere. Do four or five sets of six to eight repetitions, alternating between exercises and resting 30 seconds between sets.

ISOEXPLOSIVE PRESS-UP

Targets: Chest, Triceps, Shoulders, Abdominals

1. Get into a press-up position, hands slightly wider than and in line with your shoulders. Your body should form a straight line from your shoulders to your ankles.

2. Keep your back flat and lower your body until your upper arms are lower than your elbows. Pause, holding the 'down' position for 4 seconds.

3. Forcefully thrust yourself upwards as high as you can, so that your hands leave the floor. Catch yourself and repeat.

ISOEXPLOSIVE SQUAT

Targets: Quadriceps, Gluteals

1 Stand with your knees slightly bent and your feet shoulder-width apart.

2 Slowly lower your body as if you were sitting back into a chair, keeping your back in its natural alignment, until the fronts of your thighs are parallel to the floor, or lower. Pause, holding the 'down' position for 4 seconds. Jump as high as you can, then repeat.

ISOEXPLOSIVE BURN

To get the most out of these isoexplosive moves, hold the 'down' position of each exercise for 4 seconds, which eliminates the elasticity in your muscles. When you explode upwards, your muscle fibres will be forced to work maximally, without weights.

The 22-Minute Total Body Plan

Sculpt Your Body with 16 Essential Weight-Free Moves

You want to get back into shape, right? But between long hours at work, business travel and weekends spent frantically shuttling the kids from football practice to dance class to dentist's surgery, does anyone ever make it to the gym any more? Here's a comprehensive, total-body workout you can do any time, and just about anywhere – hotel room, home gym, garden or even in the comfort of your living room.

Daily Stretches

Spend 10 minutes every day warming up with the stretches below before your total-body workout. Hold each position for 10 seconds.

Upper-Back Stretch (p.22)
Chest Stretch (p.23)
Shoulder and Neck Stretch (p.24)
Posterior Shoulder Stretch (p.25)
Lying Iliotibial Band Stretch (p.28)
Modified Hurdler Stretch (p.29)
Groin Stretch (p.30)
Calf Stretch (p.30)

The Workout

Do the routines on alternating days. For example, do Workout A on Monday, Workout B on Wednesday and then Workout A again on Friday. The next week, do the opposite, with Workout B on Monday, A on Wednesday and B again on Friday (see chart on following page). If you're a beginner, start off with five repetitions of each exercise the first week and gradually increase the reps to 20. Do this slowly and carefully – don't push yourself too hard at first. When you're able to do 10 reps of each exercise, the workout should take about 8 to 12 minutes. The stretches should take about 10 minutes. Total workout time: 22 minutes.

Workout A

EXERCISE	BEGINNER REPS	INTERMEDIATE REPS	ADVANCED REPS
Donkey kick (p.94)	5	10	20
Dive-bomber press-up (p.69)	5	10	20
Dirty dog (p.92)	5	10	20
Lunge (p.90)	5	10	20
Side straddle hop (p.94)	5	10	20
Back extension I or II (p.74 and p.75)	5	10	20
Wide press-up (p.67)	5	10	20
Side crunch (p.86)	5	10	20
Crunch (p.79)	5	10	20

Workout B

EXERCISE	BEGINNER REPS	INTERMEDIATE REPS	ADVANCED REPS
Press-up (p.64)	5	10	20
Crunch (p.79)	5	10	20
Lunge (p.90)	5	10	20
Steam engine (p.88)	5	10	20
Elbow-to-knee crunch (p.87)	5	10	20
Prone flutter kick (p.76)	5	10	20
Hip adduction (p.93)	5	10	20
Side leg raise (p.91)	5	10	20
Diamond press-up (p.66)	5	10	20

The All-Day Workout

Build Strength and Flexibility Any Time, Anywhere

We all have time to exercise. It's the prep work that kills us. Gather your gear, drive to the gym, navigate the reception desk and locker room, warm up, cool down, stretch, shower, dress and drive home – you invest more time accommodating exercise than actually working out. But we've found plenty of exercises you can do without all that wasted time. These moves take only moments – pumping you up or calming you down – and will contribute to your overall strength, flexibility, posture and muscle. Best of all, they fit into the pockets of time hidden throughout the day – when you're between tasks at work, walking the dog or getting ready for bed. On the busiest day of your life, you'll still have time to squeeze all of them in.

LYING VACUUM

Targets: Obliques, Transverse Abdominis

■ Lie on your back in bed and try to suck your belly button all the way back to your spine. While you're at it, try to tighten up the muscles on the sides of your midsection, too. Hold for 10 seconds while you take shallow breaths. Try it three times.

BRIDGE

Targets: All Mid-body Muscles

1. Lie face-down on the floor (on a rug or mat) and prop yourself up so your weight is on your toes, forearms and hands. Your body should form a straight line from head to heels. Don't let your chest or stomach sag towards the floor. You have to tighten all your muscles to hold this position, with your abs and the muscles between your shoulder blades doing the hardest work. Again, hold for 10 seconds while breathing, and do three repetitions.

WORK YOUR ABS BEFORE BREAKFAST

When you wake up in the morning, your abs are about as visible as they're going to be all day. So take advantage: do these these abdominal exercises as soon as you wake up — you don't even have to get out of bed to do the Lying Vacuum (left).

TOWEL STRETCH

Targets: Shoulders, Triceps

1. Grab the ends of the towel with your left hand behind your head and your right hand at the middle of your back. Gently pull down with your right hand until you feel a good stretch in your left shoulder and triceps. Hold for 15 to 30 seconds. Then pull up with your left hand until you feel a stretch in your right shoulder, and hold that for 15 to 30 seconds. Repeat two or three times, slowly going from one stretch to the other. Reverse hand positions and repeat two or three more times.

SHOWER AND STRETCH

Do this stretch straight after you get out of the shower and dry off. It will help combat the tightness that develops in your shoulders when you hunch over a keyboard all day.

WALKING LUNGE

Targets: Quadriceps, Gluteals, Hamstrings

1 Lunge forwards with your right leg, then walk forwards with your left leg into another lunge step, making sure that your right foot is directly under your front knee when in the lunged position. Do a set of walking lunges for 6 metres or so, then turn round and do another set.

THE ANY TIME LUNGE

You can work the stabilizing muscles in your calves, inner and outer thighs, and mid-section by lunging instead of walking a few times a day. Do a few lunges in the morning while walking your dog or on your way to the bathroom. You can even do lunging laps around your living room while watching your favourite television show — just make sure no one sees you.

HORSE STANCE

Targets: Legs, Hips, Ankles

1 Stand with your feet shoulder-width apart and pointing forwards. Keeping your head and back straight, squat down by bending your knees and extend your arms out in front of you, palms facing each other. Hold for up to 60 seconds, then shift to the Bow-and-Arrow Stance (below).

BOW-AND-ARROW STANCE

Targets: Legs, Hips

1 Stand with your legs a little more than shoulder-width apart and extend your right foot forwards. Place your right hand on your right thigh and reach your left arm across your chest. Hold for up to 60 seconds, return to the Horse Stance (above) for 60 seconds, then repeat the Bow-and-Arrow Stance in the opposite direction for 60 seconds.

TRAINER'S TIP

The two stances shown on this page come from the world of martial arts; fighters use them to build strength and stamina in their lower bodies. These two are particularly beneficial for the muscles surrounding your knees as they increase their stability.

HIP FLEXOR STRETCH

Targets: Hips

1 Plant your left foot on an elevated surface like a bench, a step or a chair. Lean towards it, bending your left leg while keeping your right leg straight. Feel the stretch on the front of your right hip. Hold for 30 seconds, then switch legs.

TRAINER'S TIP

Stretch your hip flexors whenever you have a chance. These muscles, which sit on the front of your pelvis, can become shortened and tightened from a full day of sitting.

PART III:
The Exercises

Chest, Back and Arms

Essential upper-body exercises for total-body strength and fitness

PRESS-UP

■ **Targets:** Chest, Triceps, Shoulders

1 Get into press-up position – your hands set slightly wider than and in line with your shoulders – with your arms straight and your back flat.

2 Lower your body until your chest nearly touches the floor. Pause, then push yourself back up to the starting position.

ONE-HANDED PRESS-UP

■ **Targets:** Chest, Triceps, Shoulders

1 Spread your legs as wide as possible and move your arm towards the centre of your body as shown.

2 Lower your body until your chest nearly touches the floor. Pause, then push yourself back up to the starting position.

TRAINER'S TIP

If you're having trouble doing the One-Handed Press-up, put your hand on an elevated surface, such as a chair. This reduces the percentage of body weight you have to lift, making the exercise easier.

DIAMOND PRESS-UP

■ **Targets:** Chest, Triceps, Shoulders

1️⃣ Get into traditional press-up position, but place your hands directly under your chest with your index fingers and thumbs spread out and touching – that's the diamond.

2️⃣ Lower your body until your chest nearly touches your hands. Pause, then push your body back up to the starting position.

TRAINER'S TIP

To reap the most benefits from all your press-up pursuits, make sure you keep your back flat and your pelvis tucked in throughout the movement.

WIDE PRESS-UP

■ **Targets:** Chest, Triceps, Shoulders

① Get into press-up position, but place your hands about 12 centimetres wider than and in line with your shoulders.

② Keeping your back flat, lower your body until your chest nearly touches the floor. Pause, then return to the starting position.

ROTATION PRESS-UP

■ **Targets:** Chest, Triceps, Upper Back, Rear Shoulders

1 From the down position of a traditional press-up, raise your body. Reach your right hand towards the ceiling while twisting your torso to the right.

2 Lower your arm and then slowly lower your body, rotating your torso back so that your chest is facing the floor. Repeat on the other side.

PRESS-UP POWER

Do you know how much of your own body weight you lift when doing a press-up? The answer might surprise you. At the top position of the press-up (when your arms are extended), you're supporting about 65 per cent of your body weight. At the bottom position (when your upper arms are parallel to the floor), you're pressing about 75 per cent of your body weight. That's not so bad when you think of how much you probably bench press at the gym.

DIVE-BOMBER PRESS-UP

■ **Targets:** Chest, Front Deltoids, Triceps

1 Get into a traditional press-up position, but place your hands slightly wider than and in front of your shoulders, in line with your ears. Raise your hips and move your feet forwards as far as possible, without bending your back or legs, and place your feet beyond shoulder-width apart.

2 Move your chest down and forwards until it nearly touches the floor and your shoulders are even with your hands.

3 Pause, then push your hips down as you straighten your arms. Pause again, then reverse the movement until you've come back to the starting position.

STEP-UP PRESS-UP

■ **Targets:** Chest, Triceps, Rotator Cuffs

1 Position yourself in a traditional press-up position in front of a step or bottom stair.

2 Move your right hand onto the stair while keeping your back straight, then move your left hand onto the step. Hold this position for two seconds.

3 Remove your right hand from the step, returning it to the floor. Bring your other hand back down into the starting position. Repeat the entire sequence.

TRAINER'S TIP

Even though this press-up does not include the traditional press-up motion, it still provides a great upper-body workout by challenging your muscles to support your weight from uneven, unfamiliar angles.

STAGGERED PRESS-UP

■ **Targets:** Chest, Triceps, Back, Abdominals

1 Position yourself in a traditional press-up posture. Keep your back straight and place one hand 15 centimetres forwards, so that it is in line with your ear.

2 Lower yourself until your chest is almost touching the floor, and slowly raise yourself to the starting position. Repeat by moving the other hand forwards.

THREE-POINT PRESS-UP

■ **Targets:** Chest, Triceps, Shoulders

1 While in a traditional press-up position, place one foot on top of the other, so that the toe of the top foot is resting on the heel of the bottom foot. Your body is now resting on three points.

2 Keep your back straight and lower yourself until your chest is almost touching the floor. Slowly raise yourself to the starting position. Repeat with the other foot on top.

Y's, T's and I's

If you are the athletic type, chances are you will strain or injure your rotator cuffs — a group of muscles and tendons that surround the top of the upper arm bone and enable your arm to move from your shoulder with force and speed — at some point in your life. To avoid such injuries, you need to strengthen those muscles with these great exercises. The titles refer to the position of your arms and body as they form different letters of the alphabet. Do three sets of 10 repetitions of each.

Targets: Rotator Cuffs

▣ Lie face down on a bench and extend your arms in front of you to form a 'Y'. Keep your back straight and point your thumbs to the ceiling. Lift your arms towards the ceiling as much as you can by squeezing your shoulder blades. Although you won't move much, you'll feel a good stretch in those rotator cuffs. Lower your arms back to the starting position and repeat.

2 Next, stretch your arms, palms down, to either side of your body in the shape of a 'T'. Once again, try to lift your arms as high as you can by squeezing your shoulder blades. Lower your arms slowly and repeat.

3 Finally, pull your arms to your sides, with palms facing upwards, and form the letter 'I' with your body. Once more, raise your arms as high as you can. Slowly lower and repeat.

TOWEL CHEST FLY

■ **Targets:** Chest

1 Place your hands on either a towel or a pair of socks. Assume the traditional top press-up position, with your hands close together underneath you and your feet hip-width apart.

2 Slide your hands out to your sides as you lower your body towards the floor. Slowly slide back up. Keep your elbows slightly bent throughout the movement, and make sure that your back is straight.

BACK EXTENSION I

■ **Targets:** Lower Back

1 Lie face-down with your fingers behind your ears.

2 Simultaneously raise your upper body and legs off the floor as high as is comfortable. Pause, then slowly lower yourself back to the starting position and repeat.

BACK EXTENSION II

■ **Targets:** Lower Back

1 Lie face-down with your arms by your sides, about 5 centimetres away from your hips.

2 Simultaneously raise your upper body – including your arms – and your lower body off the floor as high as is comfortable. Pause, then slowly lower to the starting position and repeat.

BATHROOM BREAKS TO SAVE YOUR BACK

OK, so most of us spend hours on end sitting in uncomfortable desk chairs staring at computers, sealing business deals and performing a myriad of other tasks. Nothing is easier than rounding your shoulders and resting your elbows on the desk while checking out a Web site. But you have to stay clear of such posture *faux pas*. The truth is, the best posture for sitting is one that changes frequently. If your job forces you to sit at a desk, leave your chair every 20 to 30 minutes to give your back intermittent breaks from the increased stress of sitting. An easy trick that will keep you out of that chair: drink lots of water. Your bathroom breaks will give you an excuse to take your spine for a spin.

SUPERMAN

■ **Targets:** Lower Back

1 Lie face-down on the floor with your legs straight and your arms outstretched in front of you.

2 Simultaneously raise your upper body and legs off the floor as high as is comfortable. Pause, then slowly lower yourself back to the starting position and repeat.

PRONE FLUTTER KICK

■ **Targets:** Hamstrings, Lower Back, Gluteals

1 Lie face-down on the floor with your legs straight and your arms in front of you. Raise your left leg off the floor as high as you can while your right leg remains stationary.

2 Pause, then lower your left leg to the starting position. Repeat with your right leg.

Abdominals

Crunch, twist and slide your way to a strong, chiselled mid-section

SHOULDER BRIDGE

■ **Targets:** Abdominals, Lower Back, Gluteals

1 Lie on your back with your legs bent and your feet flat on the floor.

2 Push your hips up so your weight rests on your shoulders. Your body should form a straight line from your knees to your shoulders.

3 Hold this position for 20 seconds, and gradually work your way up to one minute.

TRAINER'S TIP

As your lower-body strength improves, challenge your muscles in new ways by performing this variation: straighten one leg and hold it up in the air. Start with your weaker leg in the air and give equal time to both sides.

LYING VACUUM

■ **Targets:** Obliques, Transverse Abdominis

Lie on your back and contract your lower abdominal muscles as if you are sucking in your belly button all the way back to your spine. Hold for 10 seconds while you take shallow breaths.

DON'T HOLD YOUR BREATH

Although it's natural to want to hold your breath, it's important to breathe normally when performing isometric contractions like this one. If you're having trouble with this, place your hands on your abdomen and use your fingertips to gauge the intensity of the lower abdominal muscle contractions.

CRUNCH

■ **Targets:** Rectus Abdominis, Obliques

1 Lie on your back with your knees and hips bent to about 90 degrees, and cross your arms.

2 Raise your upper body off the floor by crunching your ribcage towards your pelvis. Then lower yourself to the starting position.

TRAINER'S TIP

Where you place your hands can change the degree of difficulty of a crunch. If you can't complete the last repetition of a set, try moving your hands from behind your ears to across your chest. This displaces a portion of your weight and may allow you to do one or two more crunches, to work the muscles a little longer.

LONG-ARM CRUNCH

■ **Targets:** Rectus Abdominis, Obliques

1️⃣ Lie on your back with your knees bent and feet flat on the floor about hip-width apart.

2️⃣ With your arms stretched over your head, exhale and slowly curl your head and torso towards your knees until your shoulder blades are off the floor. Use your upper abs to raise your ribcage towards your pelvis and lift your shoulder blades off the floor. Hold for a few seconds. Don't sit up fully; your lower back stays pressed to the mat.

3️⃣ Keeping your arms in line with your head, slowly lower yourself to the starting position, inhaling as you go. Use controlled motion; don't just drop to the floor.

TRAINER'S TIPS

- Make sure your shoulder blades come off the floor each time. Don't move just your head and neck.

- Pause at the top of the movement after you've exhaled.

- To align your head properly, put your tongue on the roof of your mouth when you do crunches. It will help reduce neck strain.

CRUNCH WITH HEEL PUSH

■ **Targets:** Rectus Abdominis, Obliques

1 Lie on your back with your knees bent and only your heels on the floor. Place your hands behind your ears, but avoid pulling your head forwards.

2 Keeping your toes pointing up, slowly curl your head and torso towards your knees until your shoulder blades are off the floor. Hold for a few seconds, then slowly lower yourself to the starting position.

CROSS-LEGGED CRUNCH

■ **Targets:** Rectus Abdominis, Obliques

1 Lie on your back with your lower legs crossed on the floor. Hold your hands behind your ears and pull your elbows back as far as possible.

2 Slowly curl your head and torso towards your knees until your shoulder blades are off the floor. Hold for a few seconds, then slowly lower yourself to the starting position.

TRAINER'S TIP

For a more challenging exercise, start with your legs straight and suspended about 45 centimetres above the floor. As you curl your upper body off the floor, simultaneously raise your legs until your feet point towards the ceiling. As you bring your head and shoulders back down to the floor, lower your legs back to their starting position.

TOWEL CRUNCH

■ **Targets:** Rectus Abdominis

1 Sit on the floor with your knees bent, your feet flat on the floor and your fingers behind your ears. Set a rolled-up towel under the arch of your lower back and lie back so your head rests on the floor.

2 Raise your head and shoulders and crunch your ribcage towards your pelvis.

3 Pause, then slowly return to the starting position.

TWISTING LEGS-UP CRUNCH

■ **Targets:** Rectus Abdominis, Obliques

1️⃣ Lie on your back and raise your legs so that the soles of your feet point towards the ceiling.

2️⃣ Place your hands lightly behind your ears, elbows pointing out. Keeping your legs upright, slowly curl up and to the left.

3️⃣ Lower yourself and repeat to the right. Alternate from left to right throughout the set.

KNEE CRUNCH

■ **Targets:** Rectus Abdominis

1 Lie on your back with your knees bent and pressed together and your feet flat on the floor with your toes pointing in.

2 Place your hands behind your ears, then lift your head and curl your shoulders up off the floor. Hold and then lower.

SIDE CRUNCH

■ **Targets:** Obliques

1 Lie on your right side and cross your right arm over your chest, resting your right hand on your left shoulder. Rest your left arm on your left side, with your palm down on your thigh.

2 Crunch your left armpit towards your left hip as you raise your legs off the floor. Pause, then return to the starting position. Repeat on the other side.

FEEL THE SQUEEZE

Here's a sure way to tell whether this exercise is effective: you feel a squeeze on the side of your stomach. Unlike the traditional crunch, this exercise works your obliques.

ELBOW-TO-KNEE CRUNCH

■ **Targets:** Rectus Abdominis, Obliques

1 Lie on your back, with your left foot flat on the floor and your right foot crossed over your left knee. Keep your arms folded over your chest.

2 Crunch your upper body, twisting it towards your right side. Touch your left elbow to your right thigh. Don't move just your elbow or shoulder – make sure you twist your whole torso towards your knee. Lower yourself slowly to the starting position. Repeat on the other side after switching legs.

DON'T DO IT DAILY

Although it may be tempting to work your abs every day, they are just like any muscle group in your body: they need time to repair and rest. For best results, train them two to three times a week.

STEAM ENGINE

■ **Targets:** Hip Flexors, Entire Mid-section

1 Stand with your hands cupping your ears from behind and your feet shoulder-width apart.

2 Bend and raise your right knee while you twist your left elbow towards your knee. Crunch your left shoulder towards your right hip to make contact between the elbow and the knee. Return to the standing position. Twist to the other side.

TOWEL SLIDE

■ **Targets:** Rectus Abdominis

1 Kneel on a towel or mat on a tiled or wooden floor. Put another towel on the floor in front of you and place your hands on it.

2 Slide the front towel across the floor until your body is fully extended. Your body should look as if it's in a diving position. Slowly slide back up.

Legs

Build strong, supple muscles with this selection of lower-body exercises

THE LUNGE

■ **Targets:** Quadriceps, Gluteals, Hamstrings

1 Stand with your hands on your hips and your feet hip-width apart.

2 Step forwards with your right leg and lower your body until your right knee is bent to 90 degrees and your left knee is almost touching the floor. Raise your body back to the starting position, then repeat with your left leg.

TRY IT IN REVERSE

To really strengthen your legs, try the lunge in reverse: instead of moving forwards as in the traditional lunge, step backwards. How does it work? In a traditional lunge, your back leg gets the good stretch, while the front leg supports the movement. However, the reverse lunge forces your front leg to work throughout the entire exercise, increasing muscle use.

SIDE LEG RAISE

■ **Targets:** Outer Hips

1. Lie on your right side while supporting yourself on your right elbow. Bend your right knee, but keep your left leg straight.

2. Leading with the heel, raise your left leg about 45 centimetres, then pause. Lower the leg to the starting position. After completing a set with your left leg, change sides and repeat with the other leg.

MAXIMIZE MUSCLE USE

Want to maximize your workout? Then do your lunges before the leg raises. Why? Lunges require balance and use small muscles that stabilize your body. These muscles get tired faster and therefore should be worked before moving onto exercises that don't require their use. That way, when you do those lunges, you won't be relying on overworked muscles to keep you stable.

DIRTY DOG

■ **Targets:** Outer Hips

1. Get on your hands and knees, with your palms flat on the floor and your arms shoulder-width apart. While keeping your left leg bent, raise it out to the side from the hip.

2. Pause, then return your leg to the starting position. Repeat with the other leg.

STRONG ANKLES AND A QUICKER STEP

Improve ankle stability and increase agility with this tried and tested drill.

- Draw a line on the floor. Stand with your knees slightly bent, feet shoulder-width apart, hands in front of your body and hips back. Bend your torso forwards slightly so that you are balanced. Put your toes on the line.

- With one foot, step over the line and back repeatedly, as fast as you can, for 15 seconds. Tap your toes on the other side of the line and then return to the starting position. Repeat on the other side.

- Also, mix it up by stepping sideways, backwards, and back and forth with both feet.

HIP ADDUCTION

■ **Targets:** Inner Thighs

1 Lie on your right side, supporting your weight with your right elbow. With your right leg outstretched, place your left foot in front of your right knee, so that the left leg is bent.

2 Lift your right leg as high as you can towards the ceiling. You should feel your inner thigh working.

3 Slowly lower your leg back to the starting position. When you've finished a set, repeat with the other leg.

CURE YOUR CRAMPS

Ever overwork your legs so that they cramp up? Well, you may not have overworked them after all. Muscle cramps after a workout can be a sign of a deficiency. Your muscles need certain nutrients that can be depleted through exercise. Replace the lost potassium and magnesium in your body by grabbing a banana. Your legs will thank you.

SIDE STRADDLE HOP

■ **Targets:** Groin, Calves

1 Stand with your feet together and arms hanging comfortably at your sides.

2 Jump and land with your feet just beyond shoulder-width apart while clapping your hands together overhead.

3 Jump back to the starting position, bringing your arms back down as well.

DONKEY KICK

■ **Targets:** Hamstrings, Hip Extensors

1 Get down on your hands and knees with your arms shoulder-width apart.

2 Balance your weight on your right leg and kick your left leg back and up as high as you comfortably can.

3 Finish by pulling your knee to your chest. Repeat with the other leg.

INDEX

ALSO AVAILABLE IN THIS SERIES: